By The Grace of God I Am Alive

William Manikas

Table of Contents

Preface v

Chapter One 1

    The First Surgery 1

    Second Surgery 2

    Third Surgery 6

Chapter Two 13

Chapter Three 21

Chapter Four 28

Chapter Five 38

Chapter Six 48

Preface

This book is about my experience surviving a failed surgical procedure. It begins several years before the surgery. I was having problems moving my bowels. I had the sensation of wanting to go but nothing came out. Other times very little came out. Pain was associated with my attempts to go. I took suppositories and other laxatives but to no avail.

In 2016 I went to a specialist, Dr. Small, a gastroenterologist. He sent me to the hospital. For fourteen days I was put on a pureed diet and given laxatives. During the two weeks I had no bowel movement. In the second week I had a colonoscopy. The doctor, Dr. Bailey, who performed the colonoscopy, told me that it was difficult to get the instrument through my colon because it was twisted around. During the second week I was given a shot of Mirolax. On the thirteenth day I began to have success. Two days later I was discharged from the hospital. A surgeon, Dr. Forrest Haslup, a colleague to Doctors Bailey and Small, told me on the way out that I would be back. I was told to take a laxative, Mirolax, daily and to purchase a stool purposely made to use while sitting on the toilet. This was supposed to raise my feet about nine inches and make it easier to have a bowel movement. It worked for awhile. About a year later I began having the same problems again.

I entered the hospital and an x-ray was taken of my lower abdomen. I was prepared for another colonoscopy and was taken to the room where the procedure was to take place. Dr. Bailey was there with a surgeon. Dr. Bailey said he could not help this time because the x-ray revealed a very twisted colon. I turned to the surgeon, Dr. Quan Trang, and asked him what choice did I have? He said there was only one option and that was surgery.

For the first part of this writing I relied on hospital records. The records I received are notes by Dr. Forrest Haslup, who was my doctor after the first failed surgery during my stay at St. Joseph Hospital-North. There are thirty-one pages of notes. At a meeting with my attorney on June 28, 2018, I learned that there are different records.

There are abstracts by the doctors, complete notes and notes by nurses. My attorney did get notes of 258 pages long plus an abstract from the surgeon, Dr. Tran. My attorney's investigator said that the records received by my attorney are incomplete. Further investigation must be made to evaluate what went wrong with the first surgery. After several months I was informed by my attorney that all the records—over 5,000 pages—were received.

Chapter One
St. Joseph-North Hospital

The First Surgery

During the first week in May, 12017 I had my colostomy performed by Dr. Trang at St. Joseph North Hospital. It was a successful procedure. While there, as a patient I was Instructed how to put on my colostomy bag and to clean it. I was discharged from the hospital on May 11th. The next week I went for a follow up visit with Dr. Trang. I was informed that in three months the reverse procedure would take place. This involved connecting the colon to the rectum.

In the meantime my wife, Nancy and I took a trip to Penn Yan, New York to visit my brother for a few days. It is located in the finger lake region. From there we went to Clayton, N.Y., the Thousand Island region, and stayed there four days.

We returned home to Tampa and prepared for our trip to Europe and took an eight-day Viking

River cruise from Basel, Switzerland to Amsterdam, Netherlands. The care of my colostomy was not an obstacle. I participated in all the tours on land and most of the events on board the ship. In spite of the colostomy, we enjoyed our summer. We returned home in mid July.

Second Surgery

In late July I received a phone call from Dr. Trang's office informing me that it was time for the reverse procedure. We planned for an early August date. On August 3rd, a Thursday, I entered St. Joseph Hospital-North at 8:30 a.m. and prepared for the procedure that was to start at 10:00 a.m. Upon completion I was taken to regular room for recovery.

When I woke up, I had visitors waiting. They were Nancy, Peter and Connie, Debbie, Carole Fotopoulos and Maria Gorter. The next day I was advised to get out of bed and walk around. Nancy and I walked in the hallway and I had some pain in my lower abdomen. My nurse said it was just gas that had to get out. The next day Nancy and I took another walk in the hallway, and again I had pain. I was given morphine to alleviate the pain. Again the nurse said I had to pass gas to relieve the pain. Instead, according to the radiologist, there was an increase in gas in my abdomen. On the third day I tried to walk but the pain was so excruciating that I walked only a few steps.

During the week of June 4, 2017 I went to the records office of the hospital to get a copy my records to learn what happened to me. There is no record of what happened immediately after the first surgery and the next following six days. The records do not explain what happened to me during those six days. What happened during those days I learned from my wife, Nancy and daughter, Joanna.

An x-ray was taken of my abdomen. No definitive free air was seen. You're not supposed to have free air in the abdomen. If you do, there's a hole somewhere that isn't supposed to be there (viscus perforation, for example). Free air is not threatening but most of the time the underlying disease which produces it is life threatening.

It was then decided I should have a CT scan. During that same day I coded (flat lined) three times. When I coded the second time I was dead for fourteen minutes before I was revived. I am now here to relate my experiences.

In the attempt to revive me I had an endotracheal intubation, which often is an emergency procedure that's performed on people who are unconscious or who can't breathe on their own. **Endotracheal intubation**, usually simply referred to as intubation, is the passing a flexible plastic tube through the mouth and passed my vocal cords into the trachea (windpipe) to carry oxygen to the lungs. It is frequently performed in critically injured, ill, or anesthetized patients to facilitate ventilation of the lungs, including mechanical ventilation and to prevent the possibility of asphyxiation or airway obstruction. My pulmonologist indicated I would remain intubated for the foreseeable future. This procedure was done because I could not maintain the airway, could not breathe on my own without assistance. This was done so that I could be placed on a ventilator which pushed air into the lungs to deliver a breath to me. Moreover, once this was done, I had difficulty swallowing.

It was during this procedure when my vocal cords were damaged. One vocal cord was completely paralyzed and the other was partially paralyzed. I had a sore throat and difficulty swallowing after the procedure. Consequently, I was intravenously fed.

During those three episodes of coding, I did not see any white light or image of Christ or any angel. Maybe I am not destined for heaven or those experiences do not happen, regardless what people have said and what the Christian Church says. Maybe my heart is not open to the Triune God.

As I said above, I was out for fourteen minutes when I flat lined. I am surprised they worked that long to revive me. Usually, after five to ten minutes the doctors pronounce the patient dead. My priest was present during the attempts to revive me, and he suggested to the family the doctor should give up on me. But after fourteen minutes I came to. Surprisingly, after being out fourteen minutes I did not survive as a vegetable. The oxygen that was fed me nourished the brain adequately. After I coded three times, I was transferred to the Intensive Care Unit.

As mentioned, by priests and friends, by the grace of God I survived. I have no recollection what transpired after the second surgery. Most of the time I was in a comatose condition, and physically I was in bad shape. During the days before the third surgery out of town relatives and members of my church congregation called to find out when my funeral would take place. The word had spread that my condition was near fatal.

Medical records indicate that a CT scan revealed a clinical sepsis, and a large amount of feculent peritoneal fluid caused by a perforated viscus. The patient with a perforated viscus classically is presented with sudden and severe abdominal pain. The pain may initially have a focal location – the large bowel if perforated during surgery. Consequently, there was the presence of feces in the peritoneal cavity.

I experienced an anastomotic leak which is a breakdown along an anastomosis which causes fluids to leak. Anastomosis are used when a hollow organ such as the intestine needs to be severed and reconnected to allow fluids to flow through it, most commonly because part of the organ needs to be removed.

Third Surgery

Before I was taken down for a third surgery, Dr. Haslup notified the family that I might not make it through. He asked them what he should do. He said I had a five per cent chance of surviving. They told him to try to save me. At this time my brother, nieces, sister, daughter and other family members were present because that I was in very critical condition. Except for my aging sister, they came to my bedside.

By suction Dr. Haslup removed 3600 ml of the peritoneal fluid or 122 ounces or 15 cups. In the process he found that my anastomosis was 1 cm or almost a half an inch big. He closed the upper rectum.

Now there is a conflict in what happened during the second surgery. The medical records indicate I had a viscus perforation. However, my wife and daughter were told the suture broke between my colon and rectum. My colon was finally attached to my stomach where the previous "stoma" was located.

My family, of course, was praying for me and waiting to hear how the surgery was going. After hours in surgery, a nurse notified the family that I was being transferred to the intensive care unit (ICU).

Upon completion of the surgery I was sent to ICU. For a number of days I was in a comatose condition. However, I could hear peoples' voices. I could hear my wife talking to other family members and my daughter was at the right side of my bed talking to me.

A week later I had a tracheostomy. This involved creating an opening in the neck in order to place a tube in my windpipe below the vocal cords.The procedure involved cutting a three centimeter long transverse incision above the sterna notch. This allows air to enter the lungs. Breathing is then done through the tube, bypassing the mouth, nose, and throat. This procedure made it possible for me swallow easier.

During the first two weeks x-rays of my chest and lower abdomen were taken every day. On August 8th and 9th x-rays and CT scan were taken which revealed respiratory failure and continued underinflated lungs. The bibasilar airspace disease persisted. It is also known as alveolar lung disease, a condition of the lungs in which the air spaces are swollen and contain fluid. Pneumonia and aspiration were present. The same CTA revealed that the heart was mildly enlarged.

My cardiac pacing (pacemaker) leads were properly positioned.

A Foley catheter was placed in the urinary bladder. Another tube was placed in my stoma and emptied into another Foley. In addition, a dialysis catheter was placed in my upper right chest to prepare me for dialysis treatment. Renal retention in both kidneys was revealed. The kidneys are suppose to clean the blood and pass waste as urine. They also help filter blood before sending it back to the heart. The dialysis treatment started within a few days after the third surgery.

In addition I had pulmonary congestion and interstitial edema. Interstitial edema is an excess of fluid among cells outside blood or lymphatic vessels, which may manifest as puffiness in legs or other affected area. My legs were very much swollen and my left arm was three times larger than normal.

Another x-ray revealed the gallbladder was extended and thick-walled. A large volume of free air was still present throughout the abdomen, as well as, free fluid.

I do not remember much when I was in ICU. I do remember my friend, John Christ, coming to visit. I do not remember his second visit. I do remember that he took a picture of me with his cell phone. He put it on Face Book and it went viral. Many people, strangers, responded with prayers.

I must have come in and out of my comatose condition several times. I remember seeing Nancy and holding hands with her. She was at the hospital every day. I barely could talk then. It was in a whisper like the godfather in the movie "Godfather." Several friends came to see me but I have no memory of their visits. Tom Bougas told me he came twice. Charlie Hambos came to see me but could not see me. All he saw was machines around my bed and tubes going to all parts of my body. Other people came to visit me when I was in the ICU but I have no recollection of their visits.

One of those visitors was Father Stavros Akrotirianakis. I am told that on the Sunday after his visit, he told the congregation that there would be a funeral within a few days. When Father visited me again weeks later, he told me that he didn't think he would see me again.

I am told that my brother, Peter, sister-in-law, Connie, and Nancy stayed by my bedside for several nights. I have no recollection. Even a nurse was assigned to my room for twenty-four hours.

Because I was in a comatose condition in the first two-three weeks and I was endotracheal intubated, I could not eat or drink anything. As mentioned earlier I was living on intravenous feeding. That continued for at least nine weeks.

Soon after my third surgery I was put on a dialysis schedule. I went down for dialysis three – four times a week. It was usually four times a week. Dialysis treatment is not a pleasant one. It can last from two to four hours. My treatments were usually four hours long. It was not painful but it drains you and makes you cold. Because your blood is taken out, your body gets cold. I had blankets put on me. When the treatment is over and your clean blood put back in your body, you are exhausted.

During my stay at St. Joseph-North I was attached to many tubes. Whenever I moved any part of my body bells went off. This indicated that a tube was moved which set the bells off. A nurse had to come in, turn off the bell and adjust the tube. Whenever, I heard that bell in other hospitals I had nightmares because it reminded me of my stay at St. Joseph-North.

During the third week at St. Joseph North we were notified that the hospital could not do much for me. Maybe it was because the insurance company would not pay for additional care at St. Joseph North.

Chapter Two
Connerton Long Term Acute Care Hospital

Nancy had to find another facility for me which was covered by my insurance. Connerton Hospital in Lutz was the closest to home. So at the end of the third week at St. Joseph-North at 9:30 at night an AMC ambulance came to transport me to Connerton. The medics had to have papers completed before leaving. At 10:15 we left St. Joseph-North and arrived at the Connerton facility at 11:00 p.m.

As I was taken to my room, we passed the head nurse. She welcomed me and said that they would take good care of me. Once in the bed three – five nurses/techs came into the room and bombarded me with questions. Such as what is my birthdate, my name, my address, my wife's name etc. All this information they already had. I would stay at Connerton for a month.

I have mix feelings about my stay at Connerton. The night head nurse was a joke. She didn't do anything for me. Most of the nurses and technicians came from South America and the islands. I found the male technicians to be more responsive and compassionate.

At night I would get hot, so Nancy had to purchase a small fan for me, and it was placed close to my head. Nancy came everyday to visit me even though it took 45 minutes to drive to the hospital. Sometimes she brought mail, especially greeting cards, to me.

At both St. Joseph-North and at Connerton I was immobile. I had to be turned around in bed. I could not get out of bed to go to the arm chair or bathroom. I relied on catheters and foley bags. When you are in an immobile condition you depend on other people 100% to turn on or turn off the lights, to bath you, to change your position in bed, to get you water or crushed ice, to move you to an arm chair, to open or close the window blinds or even to help with your physical therapy. Feeling helpless, I often prayed to God to help me. He was the only one who could help me. I did not watch much TV. So I took the opportunity to pray a lot. My prayers and prayers of my friends, church congregation and family were answered by God.

When I was transferred from St. Joseph to Connerton the urinary catheter was removed, and a new one was put in position at Connerton. The nurse there was rough in slipping the catheter on. It hurt! For the duration I had it on, it was uncomfortable.

While I was being fed intravenously, I received physical therapy. It was twice a week but not aggressive. My left leg was paralyzed; my left arm and fingers had no feeling. Because I was so doped up my body was swollen very much. My left arm was three times the normal size. My left thumb and pointer finger were and are mostly numb. My three other left fingers are very sensitive to touch. My left leg could move side to side while in bed, but it could not move when the therapists stood me up. I could not raise my arms very high nor could I turn in bed. In fact, I was supported by pillows. I had pillows under my feet, under my hips, under my arms and two behind my neck and head. Being confined to a bed for so long all my muscles atrophied. They had to shift me from side to side to avoid getting bed sores by putting pillows under my hips.

Two big therapists came and we started by sitting up and sitting at the edge of the bed. I had to lift myself to a sitting position with the help of the bed railing. Sometimes I would get dizzy just sitting up. As time went by I gradually did other movements. In order to stand up two strong therapists had to hold me up because my leg muscles were very week. The next step was for me to transition to an arm chair. When the two therapists helped me up, I could move my right leg, but not my paralyzed left leg. Therefore, I could not pivot my left leg to turn around and get into the arm chair. I basically fell into it. Again I needed two people to help me out of the arm chair to get back into bed.

A speech therapist also came to check my ability to swallow regular liquids. I could not. I still remained on a no-liquid and no-food diet. To help my swallowing the therapist gave me several tongue exercises to do. The exercises were to strengthen the tongue which would prevent liquids and solid foods going down my windpipe and cause pneumonia to develop. In addition, these exercises were to improve my speaking ability.

At other times a different therapist came with rubber-like straps to exercise my arms and legs. I did not faithfully do my exercises because I was tired, especially after a dialysis treatment. Perhaps, if I tried harder my therapy, in the long run, might not have taken so long. It took a lot of energy to do my exercises. When I did not have visitors I often fell asleep. Many times my wife, Nancy told me to take a nap, but I refused because I wanted to look at her. Besides the exercises, I was tired because every two to three hours during the night I was awakened by the nurses and/or nurse assistants to take my vitals, to give me my medicines by injections, etc.

Even though Connerton was further away from Tampa, I had quite a few visitors. Nancy, of course, came every day. Friends from church came and my brother, Peter and his wife, Connie, came when they came to the Tampa Bay area in October. But first, September 24th was my birthday. Nancy planned a birthday party in my room. A birthday cake was brought into the room for the guests, but being on a no food/no drink diet I could not have a piece. My children, Tommy and Joanna came down for it, as well Peter and Connie. Others who came were Doris and Nick Andreadakis, Ron and Magda Myers and a few others from church.

One surprise visitor to see me was Father Polycarp of the Panagia Vlahernon Greek Orthodox Monastery (Williston, Fla.) outside Ocala. He wore his black cap, black robe and long black beard. A friend, Anna Mourer, from our church suggested to Father Polycarp to visit me because I was a frequent visitor to the monastery and because my priest had not seen me since the first week of my tragedy. When Father Polycarp came into the room he told Nancy it was not my time yet. God was not ready for me. He heard my confession and gave me Holy Communion.

One visitor who came was Elaine Halkias who went out and bought a vinyl writing board and black markers. Because people had a hard time understanding me when I whispered, I wrote my questions on the board. Even that was not too successful in the beginning because I could hardly write. I scribbled. Due to my atrophied muscles I had very little control over my extremities.

While at Connerton I was transported to the Florida Hospital near Florida Southern University by ambulance to have a procedure done. A "j-tube," a feeding tube was to be placed in my stomach to replace the feeding by intravenous. I was accompanied by two attractive nurses. After an hour one nurse went to find out what was the hold up. In the meantime the other nurse got a cup of coffee. She asked me if I wanted a sip. I said yes, while I was not supposed to. She got a straw and dipped into the coffee. Then I licked the straw. When I tasted that coffee I thought I was in heaven.

After another forty-five minutes the other nurse returned with a medical assistant who said the "j-tube" procedure was too risky. It might tear my stomach. So, we returned to Connerton.

A week later my doctor said they would try the "j-tube" procedure again but at the lower end of my stomach. Other doctors said it was too risky. So, it was not done. In addition to the primary doctor, I had many specialists attend to me. They included a neurologist, a cardiologist, a nephrologist, and a pulmonologist. They came two-three times a week.

During my stay at Connerton Lisa Alsina and her husband Dr. Angel, who was a surgeon at Tampa General Hospital, came to visit me. Nancy and I told Dr. Angel about the failure to do the "j-tube" procedure. He said it was a simple one and I should transfer to Tampa General Hospital. A week later I was transferred.

Chapter Three
Tampa General Hospital

Again I was transported by ambulance in the evening to Tampa General Hospital. I had a huge room overlooking the Hillsborough River and viewing the Tampa skyline. I still was on a no liquid-no food diet. Since my second operation at St. Joseph-North I was connected to oxygen. I still was connected to foley bags. I was in no condition to get up and use the bathroom. When, finally, the catheter was removed I had to use the urinal while laying bed. Because I was on a strong diuretic (Furosemide)) I frequently had to use the urinal. The Furosemide was administered intravenously instead by pill, and therefore it worked faster. So, during the night I was using the urinal almost every hour. I was taking spironolacton to remove the excess liquids from my body. My arms, thighs, legs and ankles were still very swollen. Laying in bed does not help to reduce the swelling. Activity, such as walking, helps to reduce the swelling but I was confined to the bed.

The day and night nurses and technicians were terrific. Even though my foley was connected to my stoma by tube, there were occasions when the nurses had to empty my ostomy bag. At Connerton and at Tampa General the nurses were dedicated and compassionate. It takes a special person to be in the medical field, and in my opinion it is the nurses. However, they had to come in periodically to take my vitals, administer medicine and take blood.

Tampa General is connected with the University of South Florida; therefore, it is a teaching hospital. When my specialists came in to check me out, they brought their entourage of students with them. At times I felt like being a guinea pig. Since I have been home I see some of the specialists, periodically. They include the nephrologist, neurologist, as well as my primary doctor and cardiologist.

The care I received was excellent. After the second week the "j-tube" was disconnected but still was in my stomach. I was put on a no-salt, soft food diet and could only drink honey-consistency fluids such as cranberry juice, apple juice and milk. The reason for this type of liquids was due to my difficulty swallowing (dysphagia) thin liquids. Dysphagic patients are at an increased risk for developing aspiration pneumonia because the foods and fluids that they consume may inadvertently enter their lungs.

Drinking thickened liquids can help prevent choking and stop liquid from entering the lungs. This type of liquid is not very tasty. So, I would ask the night nurses for regular ginger ale and I would sip it throughout the night. Sometimes I poured some of the ginger ale into the thickened liquid to make it taste better. Even a glass of water was of thickened consistency. The only way I could drink it, if it was cold, otherwise it tasted terrible.

To determine when I could drink regular liquids, I took a swallow test. At Connerton I had three of those tests. The technician would follow the liquids by x-ray to see if they went down the esophagus instead of going into my lungs. I failed all three swallow tests. The liquids I sipped went down into the lungs. I failed two other swallow tests later at Tampa General.

While at Tampa General my dialysis treatment stopped during the third week. It was pleasant news when the nephrologist told me. He did say that they would monitor my kidney functions in case they had to resume the treatment. By the grace of God, the treatments were not resumed.

In October, Joanna flew down for a few days to visit. One night she slept on the couch in my hospital room. In fact, that night, which was a Sunday night, we watched a NFL football game. During her many visits at the hospital and rehab facilities we watched TV, played games and talked. I looked forward to visits by my daughter and grandson. Joanna kept my spirits up with her animations.

During my four-week stay at Tampa General, I had many visitors because it was right in Tampa and not far away as Connerton. They included fellow choir members, members of my church and family. Some visitors such as Ellen Karaku, Anna and Brett Mourer, Maria Gorter and Lisa and Angel Alsina were repeaters. Other visitors included Annetta and John Alexander. I had another surprised visit by Father Polycarp from the monastery. Again I had confession and he administered Holy Communion.

When people visit the sick in hospitals they tend to bring flowers and small gifts. From my experience visitations from friends and family were more important than gifts. Having contact with the outside world and sharing information makes you feel that you still a part of it and not cut off from it. I looked forward to daily visits by my wife, Nancy. When she was not there I missed her very much.

My physical therapy continued at Tampa General. This time it consisted of two ladies. Frankly, I was not in the mood for it. One of the two therapists was a stern middle age woman. She was determined to get me out of bed, transition to an arm chair and walk. Every time she came into my room I wished I could run away. I gave her a hard time and we joked a lot. She succeeded in getting me out of bed, stand up and transition to an arm chair. With an apparatus she succeeded in getting me to walk from five to fifty steps. I placed my arms on the arm rests and the machine raised me up. Still resting on the arm rests I walked forward. Keep in mind my left leg could not move easily. While it was difficult, every step forward represented a success story. Again if I tried harder my therapy would have progressed further. Progress in therapy depends on the patient's willingness to push himself/herself harder.

While at Tampa General, Nancy and I were advised that after the fourth week I would be discharged. I still was immobile. With help I still had difficulty transitioning to the arm chair. I could not stand on my own or walk without help. I could not raise my arms more than ninety degrees up. Our options were not great. I could enter Tampa General's rehab facility for two weeks and then be sent home. However, my insurance would not pay for it. Anyway there is no way that in two weeks I could get up and move around. I would be stuck in a wheelchair and then go to an outpatient facility. That was not a good option. The second choice was to find another rehab facility that would take me for more than two weeks and accept my insurance. So, Nancy had to call and visit other rehab facilities.

Chapter Four
West Bay Rehabilitation Facility

Finally she found West Bay Rehabilitation facility in Olds Mar. Again I was transported in the evening to that facility from Tampa General, and stayed there throughout November, 2017. When I arrived my night caregiver, Anette was waiting. I was put into a room for two people. However, for several weeks I had no roommate. That was nice.

I still was immobile. As at Tampa General I was cleaned up by wipes in bed every morning. But at West By once a week I was taken to the shower room, and in a special wheelchair, I was given a shower by my night caretaker. I was taken there in a wheelchair and then transitioned to another wheelchair made specifically for showers. My caretaker washed me completely. Keep in mind I needed help to get up, and I could not stand up to wash myself. My day for taking a shower was Saturday.

Because of my immobility I could not dress myself. My caretaker had to dress me while I lay in bed. She had to put on my t-shirt, underwear and my shorts. To put on my underwear and shorts, I had to roll over to my right side and then left side. This was done several times to get them fully on. When I got back in bed after being in the wheelchair my caretaker had to take off my underwear.

Once I was able to transition from the bed to the wheel chair with the help of the caretaker, I used the bathroom to empty my bladder. However, I needed help to get up from the wheelchair, drop my pants and transition to the toilet. All the time I was holding onto the grab bar. To get up I grasped the grab bar while the caretaker pulled me up from the toilet, by pulling me up by my pants, and helped me back into the wheelchair. My legs were still very weak and I could not stand up and remain standing.

Most of the time at West Bay I was in bed, and three to four hours a day, I sat in the wheelchair. I ate my meals in my room. About a week after I arrived I started to brush my teeth in the bath room while sitting down. While in the wheelchair I went up and down the hallway. It was a good way to exercise my arms and feet. One day one of the nurses told me that sitting in the wheel chair was not good. It did not help in bringing down the swelling in my legs. So, I spent most of the time in bed. Because I could not get up and go to the bathroom by myself I had to use a urinal while in bed, especially at night.

Shortly after I arrived at this facility, my physical therapy began. A big Irishman came to my room to take me to the gymnasium. This is when my real physical therapy began. He put me in front of a bar (like parallel bars). He said he was going to help me stand up. I was taught the proper procedure for standing up. I grasped the bar and at the count of three I was to pull myself up to a standing position. Well, I could not raise myself. The therapist had a security belt on me and he pulled me up. It was difficult. Once I was up I did not have good balance. I could not stand up for more than thirty seconds. Keep in mind my muscles had atrophied from laying in bed for three months. Over a period of time I could stand for three minutes and then up to five minutes.

I received physical therapy two to three times a day five days a week. My therapy involved lifting one pound weights, raising a bar over my head, moving my arms from side to side, riding a bicycle, taking steps while sitting down, etc. With each exercise I was timed to see how long I could accomplish it. Each session was forty-five minutes long.

In time I practiced transitioning from the wheel chair to bed and back. Without this exercise I could not get out of bed. At first two therapists had to help me with this exercise. Eventually, I just needed one therapist and then I did it on my own with help of a walker to lean on.

Then one day the Irishman brought a walker to me and said I was going for a walk. Surprised, I just looked at him. He had to help me stand up. At first I took seven steps. The next day I took fifteen steps. Gradually, over a period of weeks I was able to walk seventy-five steps.

While I was doing my therapy I asked my therapist if I will be able to walk again on my own. The response was I will with a walker. That was not the answer I expected. I said I want to be able to walk again. Even at a meeting with the staff at West Bay I said I wanted to leave on my own power. They were not very positive.

In addition to physical therapy, I received speech therapy. It included doing tongue exercises to strengthen my speaking ability and to prevent food and liquids going down my windpipe. The speech therapist came three times a week between 7:30 and 8:00 a.m., during breakfast. Needless to say, I had to stop eating and my food got cold.

While at West Bay I received visitors. They included Vickie, Sunday School Director, Maria Gorter, John and Annetta Alexander, etc. Unfortunately, the room was not big enough to have more than one chair for each patient. Occasionally, my roommate's chair was borrowed to accommodate the visitors otherwise visitors had to stand.

When Annetta and John Alexander came we sat outside and talked for quite a length of time. The subject of milkshakes came up. Let me tell you about the story of the milkshake. My cardiologist, Christopher Pastore, at St.Joseph-North would periodically check in, during the first week, to see how I was doing. Remember I was on a no food, no drink diet. So, one day I said to him the first thing I would drink, when I could, would be a chocolate milkshake. We made a deal. He would buy a milkshake for both of us. So, John went across the street to the Shake and Steak restaurant and returned with two chocolate shakes. One was for me. I was familiar with this particular restaurant because one day my wife, Nancy, pushed me in the wheel chair to the restaurant. I had a chocolate shake and a grilled cheese sandwich.

Let me finish the milkshake story. In January, 2018, I had an appointment with Dr. Pastore. He had forgotten about our deal. He told me that on the next visit I should remind his staff about our deal. So during my next visit I reminded the office staff about the milkshake deal. While Dr. Pastore was examining me, one of his office girls came in with two chocolate milkshakes.

Another visitor was a fellow choir member and colleague at Hillsborough Community College who also was a guitarist. It was John Demas who came one evening and for almost an hour played his guitar for me.

A week after I was at West Bay I got my first roommate. He was unbearable. He yelled out during day and night. It was difficult to sleep. He must have been a minister or very religious. He would yell out "praise the lord" with his loudest voice. Other times he would yell out his wife's name and asked for her. When my daughter and her family came down to visit me during Thanksgiving, they witnessed this yelling.

They came on a Thursday and left Saturday. Before they came to the rehab facility, they stopped at Cracker Barrel and purchased dinner for their family and me. We went to a visiting room and ate our Thanksgiving dinner.

While at West Bay, I still had the "j-tube" and the dialysis device in me. About the third week, I was taken to Meese Hospital in Clearwater and they were removed. It was an outpatient procedure. When the "j-tube" was removed, it left a hole in my upper abdomen, but a bandage covered it. It would take six to seven months before the holed healed.

While at West Bay I had my first outing. Nancy decided to take me outside in the wheel chair for the fresh air and sunlight. Across the street was a Steak and Shake Restaurant. She pushed me on the sidewalk and across a wide street to the restaurant. I had a chocolate milkshake and a grilled cheese sandwich. It was a welcomed change.

After four weeks at West Bay my insurance stopped paying for my stay at the rehab facility. So, Joanna, Stephen and Nancy were trying to find another rehab facility for me. Nancy mentioned Brighton Gardens which she had seen when visiting someone there. She said it was a very nice place. It was a combination assisted living and rehab facility. So, Friday, the day after Thanksgiving, Joanna and Stephen checked it out. They liked it too and proceeded to sign a contract for me to go there. The next day Nancy visited two other facilities closer to home, and she liked both of them. But it was too late to make the changes.

It took about a week to process the papers. The insurance stopped paying, so my therapy came to an end while I was waiting to go to Brighton Gardens' assistant facility. In the meantime I got a new roommate. He was not better than the previous one. He entered West Bay in the evening. When his brother prepared to leave, the new roommate wanted to leave too. After his brother left, he tried to get out of bed. He wasn't supposed to. I told him to stay in bed, otherwise he would fall. After six tries he got out of bed. He used the food table as a crutch, and walked down the hall butt-naked.

Chapter Five
Brighton Gardens

Finally I was transferred to Brighton Gardens, my last stop before coming home. I would be there four and a half months. I arrived on December 5, 2017. I was taken to my apartment on the second floor, room 207. It consisted of two rooms, a bathroom, and a foyer with a refrigerator and cabinet. The bedroom had a bed, a night table and a big dresser.

I arrived at Brighton in the afternoon, and I was greeted by the staff and my caretaker. Unable to walk independently, I immediately sat in the wheelchair. For three and one half months, I alternated between the bed and wheelchair. Arriving without adequate clothes, I had to call

Nancy to bring me shorts, pants, underwear, socks, shirts, etc.

That evening I was taken down for dinner and introduced to my table mates. The meal portions were small but more than adequate. Residents could ask for more food, deserts and drinks. After dinner I went back to my apartment. That night, my evening caretaker, Tim, assisted me in getting undress for bed and helped me get into bed. Since I was still immobile he had to lift my legs onto the bed. I slept on my back all night. I could not turn to either side until early March.

My day caretaker was Ogdin. She was Haitian, as many caretakers were. She was big and strong. Until early March she woke me up every morning, helped me dress, shaved me once in awhile and then take me to the bathroom. During the first two months she wheeled me down to breakfast, and I wheeled myself to my apartment afterwards. By the second week in February I wheeled myself to all the meals and back again.

Two weeks after I arrived, my physical, occupational and speech therapy started. Ken was the physical therapist for awhile and he worked to strengthen my ankle, thigh, leg and abdomen muscles. In February he started me on the walker. At first I walked down one third of the hallway, then half way, then the whole length. I eventually walked down the whole length of the hallway and back to my room.

The exercises I did to strengthen my lower extremities involved, at first, doing them while sitting in the wheel chair. Eventually, Ken gave me new exercises to do while standing with the walker. Since my legs and thighs were very weak, I had to strengthen them before I could walk at a normal speed with the walker.

My occupational therapist was Paul who at first worked on strengthening my arms by pulling on straps. Since I could not raise my arms, we worked on exercises to raise and extend my arms. We also worked on transitioning to the bed from the wheelchair and back. In addition, he taught me how to dress and undress myself with a device made just for that purpose. Then he taught me how to get up from the wheelchair and sit on the toilet with the help of the grab bar. This involved pushing my pants down to the ankles and then pulling them up afterwards.

I sat on the toilet seat just to urinate. I could not stand to empty my ostomy bag. My caretaker had to do that while I sat on the toilet. As my legs got stronger, Paul directed me to stand, empty and clean the ostomy bag. From March and afterwards I was able to do this by myself. Before Paul finished with me as a therapist, he taught me how to use a pulley device to raise my arms and to swing them backwards. This pulley device came home with me in April, 2018.

The therapist, Ken, was replaced by Laurie at the end of February. Before Paul discharged me from occupational therapy he told me I was well enough to drive a car since my right leg and right arm were normal again. Ken and Paul were the best physical and occupational therapists I had. They knew how hard to push me and when to stop to rest a few minutes. As my therapy continued they were impressed on how well I was doing. Laurie got me to the point where I discontinued using the walker, and relied on the cane.

Melissa was my speech therapist throughout my therapy period. She was terrific. She gave me additional tongue and voice exercises to strengthen my swallowing and voice. Melissa was able to get me a swallow test at St. Joseph-North, and I passed it with flying colors. A week after the test I was back drinking normal liquids.

During my four and a half months at Brighton Gardens I experienced good times and bad times. When I first arrived I had a very thirsty feeling. At each meal I drank four eight-ounce glasses of liquids. They were water, milk, orange juice, cranberry juice or apple juice. I didn't realize the harm I was doing to myself. By January I was hard time sleeping because I was at first breathing hard and then I had a difficult time breathing. The nurse was notified and came to my room. Right away he realized I had to go to the hospital emergency room. The first responders were notified and they quickly came to Brighton and to my room. They immediately administered oxygen and I felt better. But I was transported to Tampa General Hospital, at my request. I had congested heart failure. I have weak heart function which results in a congestion of blood flow in the lungs and throughout the body. The former results in shortness of breath, while the latter results in swelling of the legs and possibly the hands. I was in the hospital for six days.

I then reduced my intake of liquids to three eight-ounce glasses per meal. Again I had the breathing problem and ended up at St. Joseph-North for three days at the end of January. I had congested heart failure again. I reduced my intake of liquids again, but ended up in the emergency again in February, just overnight, with the same problem.

Afterwards, I strictly adhered to two glasses of liquids at meal time. Since I have been home I follow the same regiment. In addition to limiting my liquid intake, exercises, as well as walking, keeps the swelling down. Because I was getting congested heart failure so easily, the doctor ordered weekly chest x-rays for two months to check on the fluid in my lungs.

One day while I was sitting in the wheelchair in my apartment, I dropped my cell phone which slid under the bed. I got to my knees to try to retrieve it, but I could not reach it. I tried to get up but my legs were not strong enough to hold me up. I pressed on the call button many times. After ten minutes Ogdin, my caretaker, came to help me. She did not pull me up. She told me to grasp the walker with one hand and push myself up by pushing down on the bed. It worked. When I related this incident to Ken, the physical therapist, he taught me the proper way to get up.

While my wife visited me almost every day, my daughter, Joanna, came down with my grandson, Thomas, from Virginia five times. In January, she came down alone for two weeks, leaving her family behind and taking time off from work. While visiting me she went out and bought additional furniture for my apartment. They included two chairs, three small tables, one floor lamp and two table lamps.

While here, Joanna started to take me out for breakfast, or lunch or dinner or just rides. I had to be wheeled to the car. We took the wheelchair with us for me to use once we got to a restaurant. It was a welcomed change. After Joanna left, Nancy took me out many times. Several times she took me home for the day. By this time I was able to use the walker. One day we even visited a friend at another rehabilitation facility.

As I have written earlier having visitors is more important than having flowers or candy.

With visitors you are interacting with people and keeping up with friends and family.

To occupy the residents at Brighton Gardens, programs were provided. They included singers, small bands, storytellers, exercise sessions, pingo, puzzles and movies. I attended several good movies.

The first two weeks at the assisted living facility, I went to my apartment after dinner. The program director, Kim, encouraged me to play pingo. In the third week I started going, and soon I was going every time (five times a week) they offered pingo. I met quite a few friends there. They were El, Clyde, Flo, Mary, Joann, Annalorie, and Prudent. It was very enjoyable and I won some money. After I left Brighton Gardens, I returned several times to visit my friends and play pingo.

In the living room there was a table with a puzzle on it. Anyone could work on the puzzle. I ignored it during the few months I was there. By mid-February I would sit at the table for a half an hour and put pieces together. By the end of February I would spend an hour after breakfast everyday and an hour after pingo putting the pieces together. I quickly got a reputation as the man who worked on the puzzles and usually finished them within forty-eight hours. As soon as a puzzle was completed, Kim put a new one on the table.

Brighton Gardens also put on "Family Nights" before a holiday. One such "Family Night" was before Christmas. My family attended. They included my wife, Nancy; my brother Peter and his wife Connie; and their daughter Martha with her husband, David. We had a good time eating and drinking. The dining room and parlor were filled with many family members of the residents.

By the end of February my physical therapist, Laurie, suggested I go home to save money and have home care therapy at home. So, my daughter and I officially notified the staff at Brighton Gardens that April 15th was my last day there and I would leave to go home. I left on April 10th and resumed my therapy until the end of April when Baycare Homecare discharged me.

Chapter Six
Home at Last

Being home again is a great feeling. Now at home my wife became my care taker. She wanted to help in many ways such as taking a shower, getting dressed, making breakfast, etc. I told her if I didn't do these things myself, it would delay my road onto recovery. In April grab bars were put into our bathrooms and bathtub and a chair was put into the bathtub.

Even though Paul, my occupational therapist, told me in March I could drive a car, when I got home Nancy insisted I wait awhile. I wanted to drive the car but Nancy did not let me for about ten days. When I started to drive Nancy would not get in the car with me for several weeks.

As soon as I arrived home I continued my exercises, but my balance was not good and my stamina was weak. At the end of May I visited my primary doctor and told her my concerns. She prescribed more home care therapy. So, in early June it was renewed and continued until mid-

September. The therapist, Lauren, worked on my balance and stamina. She explained that even after discharging me, it would take more exercises and time to build up my stamina.

Every day I feel improvement. My balance is improving but I will still need a cane to walk because of my bad knee. In time, with exercises my stamina will improve, too. Before my misfortune in August, 2017 I walked with a cane. I will still walk with a cane, but I have accomplished my final goal which is the ability to walk again.

When one comes face to face to a near death experience, you have to think positively and struggle to survive. In the first two months my aim was survival. It was doing this period I turned to God and asked for His help. For the next six and a half months, while in institutions, my aim was to improve my mobility. I gradually went from a wheelchair to a walker to a cane. While I am at home I still receive Homecare to improve my stamina.

This success in surviving and regaining movement in all my extremities would not have been accomplished without God's help who answered the prayers of my family, friends and strangers. Now when I attend church I am more attentive to the prayers of the services.

By the Grace of God I Am Alive.

www.ingramcontent.com/pod-product-compliance
Lightning Source LLC
Chambersburg PA
CBHW030509220526
45464CB00006B/2729